TURN RIGHT, GOOD MOON
CONVERSATIONS WITH A DYING MOTHER
L.E. MOORE

TO OUR SISTER, THE CONSTANT ONE, WITH GRATITUDE AND THANKSGIVING

Published by Tonewood Knoll Pty Limited
P.O. Box 809
Double Bay, NSW 1360 Australia

Distributed by Good Moon LLC, P.O. Box 515, Waite Park, Minnesota, U.S.A 56387

Second printing: April 2014
ISBN 978-0-9924504-0-3
ISBN 978-0-9924504-1-0 (iPad App)

National Library of Australia Cataloguing-in-Publication entry:

Moore, Leslie Ellen, author.
Turn right, good moon : conversations with a dying mother /
L. E. Moore.
ISBN: 9780992450403 (paperback)
Mother--Death--Psychological aspects.
Terminally ill parents--Home care--Anecdotes.
Palliative treatment--Anecdotes.
Last words.
Farewells.
155.937

Printed in Minneapolis, Minnesota, U.S.A.,
by As Soon As Possible, Inc., 3000 France Avenue South,
Saint Louis Park, MN, U.S.A., 55416, with thanks to George West and his team.

This book is set in Minion Pro. It is printed on acid-free paper.

We acknowledge with gratitude permission to reprint the following works or selections therefrom:

♦ Selection from "Manido Great Spirit Moon," by Joseph Bruchac, from *No Borders* (Holy Cow! Press, 1999), © 1999 by Joseph Bruchac. Used by permission of Holy Cow! Press.

♦ "Silent Winter's Night" © 2011 by Warren Moore.

♦ Selection from *Goodnight Moon* © 1947 by Harper & Row. Text © renewed 1975 by Roberta Brown Rauch. Illustrations © renewed 1975 by Edith T. Hurd, Clement Hurd, John Thacher Hurd and George Hellyer, as Trustees of the Edith & Clement Hurd 1982 Trust. Used by permission of HarperCollins Publishers.

Good Moon: It's so peaceful. There should be more written about this.

The Fledgling: Written about what?

Good Moon: About dying like this, at home.

The Fledgling: Is it good?

Good Moon: It's wonderful.

To Bev
with all good wishes
Leslie Moore
August 2014

Introduction

ONCE UPON A TIME – not in my time, not in your time, but in someone's time – there was a woman, eighty-two years young, who wanted to die from Death. Her name was Good Moon.

What would it be like, she wondered, to follow the Old Ways? To forgo food and, finally, water? To die at home surrounded by children, grandchildren and extended family as the ancestors had done for thousands and thousands of years?

We, the authors of this story, are Good Moon's children. We certainly didn't plan to tell the story of our mother's death. The story simply happened to us, around us and through us, as stories sometimes do.

It all started when the Artisan, Good Moon's daughter, arrived at the home where her mother was dying. Before she knew it, she was writing. She wanted to capture Good Moon's voice, to create a memory that would outlive Death.

The Artisan's siblings saw her with a journal, and they asked her to write for them as well. The Artisan listened and wrote for her sisters and brothers – the Constant One, the Laughing One, the Witness, the Penitent, the Driver, and the One from Far Away.

Would Good Moon approve? We didn't know, and so we told her that we were writing down her words. When we asked for her blessing, she gave it readily, and then she gave us something else. She suggested that more needed to be written about dying at home, and that idea – her idea – became this little book.

We didn't realise that reaching for our mother's words and recording her final days would alter our own relationship with Death.

Good Moon never said, "Explore with me," but that is what she wanted. She was curious. We were, too. We looked at Death. We held it, flipped it, shook it, rattled it. We plucked at it and bounced it on the floor. We held it like a shell against our ears.

Dying, that thing "out there," hidden behind hushed doors, entered the room and made itself at home. We could feel it gliding through our fingers, brushing past our hair, grazing on our arms.

The journey we shared was alive with nature, myth and spirit; with the owl, the wolf and the raven; with the sun and the moon and the stars of the Milky Way; with the ancestors – Native Americans and Africans from the Sans tribe; with music, poetry and stories; and with the deep, practical wisdom of the nurses from Hospice, who taught us how the dying die.

Above all, our journey was guided by the moon. Our mother, during her life, had held the moon deep in her heart, living in harmony with its phases. In the last decade of her life, she had edited an anthology of art and writings about the moon.

Perhaps it is not surprising, then, that Good Moon learned of her final illness on the night of a full moon in November. She died a month later, the day after a full moon in total eclipse.

Looking back, we think she may have planned it that way.

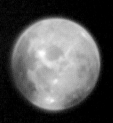

BEFORE
DARK MOON

THE YEAR THAT ENDED WITH HER DEATH was a rich one for Good Moon. In January, she travelled to Antarctica, and in May, she canoed in the land of the voyageurs. In July, she went skydiving with her grandchildren, parachuting toward earth in the arms of her instructor. In August, she competed in the local dragon boat races, and in October, she took a long hike by the great lake near her home.

In early November, Good Moon went into the hospital for a minor operation. Three days later, she gazed at the full moon, November's Dark Moon, and reflected on the call she had received from her doctor.

The Artisan lived far away from her mother, in a land where kookaburras laugh and children splash in aqua seas. In early November, she opened a short note from Good Moon. The Artisan read the note again and again, but she couldn't get past her mother's words: "In a nutshell, the biopsy was positive for ovarian cancer."

Good Moon had agreed to surgery, but she had wrestled with the decision. She had always felt that, once in her eighties, she wouldn't "clog up the healthcare system." She wrote:

> However, the choice is not so simple. By not having the surgery you are still a drain – as organs shut down and you still need care. But I have nothing to complain about. I have had such a wonderful life – so why not me as concerns cancer?

Was Good Moon facing death? If so, what were her thoughts about what was coming next?

You know how I am attracted to adventures. Well, this will be a humdinger!

In the middle of November, Good Moon walked with her granddaughter down to the shore of the great lake near her home. They sat on the rocks and were watching the waves when an arc of white flashed overhead.

Good Moon looked up. "It's a snowy owl."

The bird circled once and settled on the rocks. He wrapped his giant wings around his frame, and then he turned his head and amber eyes and fixed them on Good Moon.

There they sat, taking each other's measure, and the granddaughter wondered at the bond between the woman and the bird. When at last the owl took flight, his wings caught the light and the dark of the waves below.

After a time, Good Moon turned toward home, but over the coming days, she kept remembering the owl. She told her daughters about Wahikokohas:

His feathers make patterns
of life and death.
His wings are the shape of stories.

She saw in him a messenger, a harbinger of death.

Near the end of November, Good Moon went in for surgery. She woke to the news that her cancer had spread and that her illness was terminal. She discussed the options for treatment and decided against all of them. She chose a course of palliative care.

Good Moon told her daughters that she wanted to follow the ways of the Sans tribesman, one of the oldest peoples in the world. When their elders sense the approach of death, they stop eating and drinking.

"The people make a nest in the grass," said Good Moon, "and the elders lie down and die."

By the last day of November, Good Moon was out of the hospital. She went to the home of our sister, the Constant One, a trained nurse.

Good Moon was given the sun room, a bright, peaceful room with a comfortable bed. She looked through a broad row of windows onto the winter grass and the trees across the street.

Good Moon appeared to be feeling better. She was able to walk, and she ambled into the living room, sat in a chair, and admired the Christmas tree. She drank some chicken broth, and she ate two bites of a boiled egg and half a soda cracker.

And then, at midnight, she began to vomit. Twenty four hours later, she was near death.

On the first day of December, a voice called to the Artisan from the depths of her soul. "Get on a plane, and come home now."

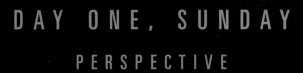

DAY ONE, SUNDAY

PERSPECTIVE

TWO DAYS LATER, on a Sunday in early December, the Artisan arrived at the home of the Constant One.

Good Moon was in the sun room, lying on a bed near the window. Her face was still brown from the summer sun, and her hair fell in wisps of silver around her forehead.

Our sister, the Laughing One, leaned over Good Moon and placed an ice chip in her mouth.

Good Moon focused her eyes on the Laughing One's nose as if she were solving a difficult problem.

"Your nose is beautiful from the right angle," said Good Moon. "I wish your husband could see it from this view."

"My husband is always looking down on my nose," said the Laughing One.

Good Moon continued, undeterred. "From this perspective, your nose is beautiful."

Then Good Moon turned to the Artisan. "Your hair."

Of course, thought the Artisan. My hair. There are things in life you can never get right.

"You can wear your hair this way into your sixties and seventies," said Good Moon.

Fifty years, thought the Artisan. Three hundred different hairstyles. "Have I finally gotten one that works?"

Good Moon nodded. "Yes."

The Artisan sat with her mother until the sun dipped behind the trees. She rubbed Good Moon's hair as if she were stroking a sleepy cat, and she thought about her mother's words.

What do the dying say to us? That there is a beauty in the living that only the dying can see?

Over the coming week, we learned that Good Moon's conversations were full of a rich liquid. The containers that held her words were heavier than ours. They needed to be. Her words were dense, and they held more meaning. The vibrations came to us like the beating of wings. They were stronger than anything we had heard before.

Later that day, our brother, the Penitent, sat with Good Moon in the growing dark.

He leaned over his mother's small, brown face. "You look like a little fawn. You're asleep on a bed of ferns in the midst of a redwood forest."

Good Moon raised her hand and touched her son's cheek.

"A whisker rub," said the Penitent.

"It's wonderful," said Good Moon. "I wish we had done this years before."

The Penitent heard someone singing. "You – are – so – beautiful – so – beautiful – to – me."

He listened, and when he realised that the voice was his own, his eyes filled with tears. He lowered his head to say goodbye, and as he did, he brushed Good Moon's lips with a kiss.

Then he turned away, as he always did.

Good Moon laid her hand on his cheek. "Please come back."

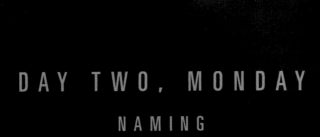

DAY TWO, MONDAY

NAMING

AT MIDDAY on Monday, a holy man from the Dakota tribe came to visit our mother.

The Healer invited us to join him in a ceremony, and it was here that our mother, after eighty-two years of living, came to know her name.

A large, full man, with hair the colour of midnight and a voice rich with the timbre of the Old Songs, the Healer sang in Dakota over our mother. He sang of living and of dying, of the journey to the ancestors and of the destination, the Milky Way.

As the ceremony unfolded, the Artisan felt a darkness so palpable that she could almost touch it, almost glimpse the edge of the mysteries. The song carried her past the sun and the moon and the stars, out to the edge of all known things, to the place where the ancestors waited, arms outstretched.

Our mother closed her eyes and listened, and at the end of the song, she asked for a translation. She was given words of blessing, simple words, deep words, words of great comfort and possibility.

And then the naming. "Wastĕ Hanyetuwi," said the Healer.

Our mother cocked her head. The syllables were unfamiliar.

The Healer spoke again, slowly. "Wash – tay – Hahn – yeh – too – wee." He paused to let the sounds sink in. "Your name means 'Good Moon.'"

"Ahhhhhh." Good Moon breathed out, and then she smiled. "Good Moon," she murmured. "Good Moon."

She tried to say her name in Dakota. "Wash –" she began, and then she faltered. The name was right, but the syllables – they were hard for her.

"Wash – tay," said the Healer, and Good Moon followed him. "Wash – tay."

And then, as if she were an echo, "Wash – tay, Wash – tay, Wash – tay."

"Hahn – yeh – too – wee," said the Healer.

"Hahn – yeh – too – wee," said Good Moon. "Hahn – yeh – too – wee."

Good Moon looked up at the Artisan. "You'll need to write down the name so I can work on it."

"I'll do that," said the Artisan.

"You don't need to worry," said the Healer. "When you reach the Milky Way, the ancestors will know who you are. Good Moon knows her name."

As he left, the Healer gave a final set of directions. "Wasté Hanyetuwi, there's only one thing you need to remember. When you reach the Milky Way, turn right. Just that – turn right."

"I will," said Good Moon.

From then on, we called her "Good Moon." The name gave us a sense that she already held the spirit of an ancestor. And how she loved her new name.

"Mom" fell away. She was still our mother, but the new name, "Good Moon," meant that she was more herself, not simply a relation, a mother to her children.

She followed her own orbit.

18

That afternoon, the Artisan spent a few minutes with Good Moon. The sun room was bright with flowers, with photographs and cards and a white coverlet on the bed, with so much light and life.

The Artisan felt two worlds, one behind the other. Behind the light was a veil of dark, a world of thick, strange greys, unbounded by space and time. A world where the ancestors, ancient and beyond all things, waited at the end of days.

And where was Good Moon, the Artisan wondered. In the light? In the dark? In the shadows in between?

The Artisan moved her chair closer to the bed. She was worried about her sister. As a nurse, the Constant One was a consummate professional – Good Moon was receiving the best of care. But as a daughter, the Constant One was awash in grief. Could Good Moon help?

"The Constant One," said the Artisan. "To her, you are irreplaceable."

Good Moon nodded. "I will let her know that she can go on."

"Please tell her that," said the Artisan.

It was quiet for a minute or two.

The Artisan reached for her mother's hand. "Let me hold your hand."

"I need to sleep," said Good Moon.

The Artisan moved her hand away.

Late that night, the Laughing One sat with Good Moon. She thought about the Sans tribesmen making a nest of grass for their dying elders.

She called for the Constant One, and together they prepared a nest. They chose three prayer shawls and a blanket, all in the colours of moonrise – periwinkle, a rich plum and a royal purple laced with gold. They swaddled Good Moon so that all they could see were a brown face, grey-green eyes, and spiky, feathered hair.

The Laughing One leaned over and whispered, "Good night, my little chickadee."

Good Moon smiled. "I love that name." And then she chirped, "Chick – a – dee – dee – dee – dee – dee."

In the deep hours of early morning, Good Moon's daughters turned their mother toward the window.

The moon had passed the third quarter and was waxing toward full. As light poured onto the bed, Good Moon murmured, "It's so beautiful."

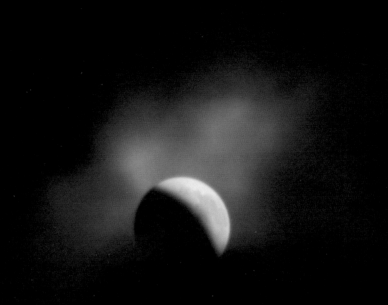

DAY THREE, TUESDAY

VOYAGEUR

EARLY TUESDAY MORNING, the Constant One sat in the living room and tried to imagine the day ahead.

Even though all of us cared for Good Moon, our sister, as a nurse, shouldered the responsibility for our mother's well-being. She was the gatekeeper, the one who balanced Good Moon's need for rest against the needs of her family and friends.

The Constant One supervised Good Moon's personal care and exercise, handled her bodily fluids, and made sure that she was turned every two hours. She managed Good Moon's respiratory function and monitored the integrity of her skin. She worked with Good Moon to control her pain and to keep her as comfortable as possible. She communicated with the nurses from Hospice, carried out their protocols and followed the doctor's orders.

That Tuesday morning, for a few precious minutes, our sister laid her constancy aside. No longer the keeper of the lamp, she became, once again, Good Moon's daughter. She sat in the grey light of dawn and cried for the mother who was leaving her.

When she was done, she stood up and turned toward the sun room, once more the keeper of the gate.

Good Moon's lawyer arrived at midday. He wanted to make sure that she was still of sound mind.

"What is your name?" asked the lawyer.

Good Moon gave her name.

"Do you have any children?"

"No."

The daughters gazed at their mother in astonishment. The lawyer looked concerned. "You – uh – you don't – have any children?"

"No," said Good Moon. "Not with my current husband."

We doubled over laughing. Ah, she was a sly one, that Good Moon.

The lawyer went on to read the will.

When he was finished, Good Moon said, "You've skipped one part."

The lawyer reviewed the document. "So I have. We can't put one over on you, can we?"

At the end of the reading, Good Moon signed her name. She held the pen and wrote with the utmost care, each word a recollection of her life.

The Artisan looked at the signature. Her mother's first name was still in this world, aligned with the words in the will. But the rest of her name slanted upward, as if ascent were imminent, words already in flight.

◆◆

In the afternoon, the Penitent sat in the sun room.

Good Moon was smiling. "I'm imagining you in a house with a garden and a dog, and with a girlfriend – or a roommate –"

The Penitent laughed. "Let's go with the girlfriend."

"A girlfriend, then."

Good Moon raised her hands. "I want to touch the back of your head."

The Penitent leaned over the bed, and Good Moon rubbed her palms against the grey stubble of her son's hair.

"It kind of feels like Velcro," said the Penitent.

After dinner, Good Moon's children and grandchildren met in the sun room to exercise her limbs. Each night, we took her on an imagined journey to awaken the circulation in her arms and legs.

"How would you like to travel this time?" asked the Laughing One. "By canoe? Or maybe by kayak?"

"By bicycle," said Good Moon.

As we lifted her arms and legs in a slow, rich undulation of dance, the Artisan told the story of her journey.

"Good Moon rode through a midnight world that blossomed under the light of the moon. Her face and hair radiated moonbeams, and the spokes of her bicycle whirled in rays of silver.

"She rode north along the shores of the great lake, through villages and towns, past the great boats and piles of ore. On the way, she stopped in a town of artists and galleries where she bought a painting of a woman who lived by moonlight.

"She rode through lands held by the Dakota tribe. She greeted the living and longed for the ancestors at the edge of the universe.

"She rode until she came to a town that, in days of old, had drawn the voyageurs from the deep north, their canoes piled high with furs.

"There she left the road and cycled down to the shores of the great lake."

The Artisan paused. Good Moon had chosen a land craft, and before her all was water. There was nowhere else to go.

But the journey wasn't done. The breath of the ancestors entered the room, and the Artisan heard more words, unplanned words, slipping past her lips.

"Good Moon looked out – beyond the land and across the waves toward an island hidden by mist.

"The colour of the world began to change. Good Moon rode across the waves, and as the island came into view, the moon began to set.

"She pulled onto the rocky shore, laid her bicycle on a bed of lichen, and gazed toward the forest. There, waiting for her, were a timber wolf and a snowy owl.

"The wolf sat in the shadow of the trees, grey, thoughtful, silent.

"The owl sat on the rocks, white wings folded, resting, alert. Alive to his next visitor.

"Good Moon saw the wolf and the owl, and she smiled."

Then the world went dark, and there was nothing more to tell.

Good Moon breathed out. "Ahhhhhh." She looked up at the Artisan. "I would like you to write down the story so you can tell it again and again." And more slowly. "I would like you to tell me the same story tomorrow night."

Yes, thought the Artisan, but when she tried to speak, the words caught in her throat. She couldn't tell the story again. Her mother had gone beyond the story, well beyond.

Good Moon had left the continent. She had settled far from the land of the living, on an island where Death was watching in a still, grey form, and where Death's voyageur was lingering, quiet, snow-winged, waiting.

Good Moon was miles ahead of us. She had thought about dying long before the diagnosis, and she knew what she wanted. Choice.

She was in her eighties – she knew that Death would come. But if she had the chance, she would choose the manner of her departure.

Choice. We saw what it looked like. Choice took courage, an acknowledgement that the end was – well – now. Not some other time. Now. Right now.

We marvelled at the thought of choice. The power of it. The peace of it. The dignity. The comfort.

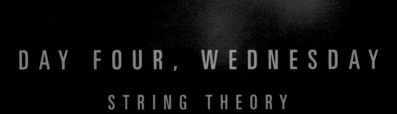

DAY FOUR, WEDNESDAY

STRING THEORY

ON WEDNESDAY, Good Moon woke at sunrise. She turned to the Constant One and said, "I'm going to sleep, and then I'm going to work."

"Your work is done," said the Constant One. "You're on vacation."

Later that day, Good Moon's daughters spoke about her plans. We were confused. What work remained? Was it the work of dying?

After breakfast, the Artisan spoke to Good Moon. "We're writing down the things you're saying to us. They're wonderful words. We're laughing, and we're happy."

Good Moon smiled. "That's so good."

"Each time you go to sleep, I will say to you, 'Good night, Good Moon.'"

"I love that book," said Good Moon.

Mid-morning, the Penitent sat with Good Moon and told her a story.

"When I was a little boy, you came back from a trip and gave me a toy elephant. It was made of grey clay, and I liked the feel of it in my hand. It was my favourite toy.

"One day, I dropped it on the floor, and one of its legs broke off. I was so upset. I brought the leg and the little elephant to you.

"You held the elephant in one hand, and with the other, you held the leg up to the light. Then you went to the cupboard and pulled out a box of toothpicks and some glue.

29

"With a needle, you bored two tiny holes, one in the elephant and the other in the leg. You placed a drop of glue in each hole, and then you took a toothpick, broke off a piece and put one end in the leg. A splint! You pushed the leg back in place and held it while the glue dried. When you were done, the leg was as good as new."

Mother and son were quiet as the story floated through the room. A young boy. A young mother. A toy elephant. A shattered leg.

"That's a wonderful story," said Good Moon.

The Penitent watched the memory disappear, and then he wound himself back to the present. There they were, a mother and a son, a man in middle age and a woman on her deathbed.

"I have carried that story with me all these years – the care you took with that little boy." The Penitent wiped his eyes. "What you did meant so much to me. Thank you."

"It's the little things that are most important," said Good Moon.

Shortly before midday, the Constant One stood outside the sun room. She took a deep breath and wiped the tears from her eyes. Good Moon was ready for the next phase of her journey. She needed a nurse to help her on her way.

The Constant One entered the room. "Good Moon, are you ready?" Her voice was soft and low.

"I'm ready," said Good Moon.

"No more water?"

"No more water."

The Pastor arrived at noon. The Constant One called Good Moon's children and grandchildren into the sun room, and we formed a circle around the bed.

The Pastor opened a small volume, turned to a well-worn page and read a blessing for the dying.

Images of guidance, a kind instruction, settled on the room. Good Moon was asked to look at us, to hold our faces in a warm embrace. We, in turn, were asked to speak to her, to give her words, our lives, our stories.

She looked at us, and we called back. Imprint. Echo.

In the afternoon, we sat around the dining room table. The nurse from Hospice had checked on Good Moon, and now she was working with us, explaining how the dying die.

She described how dehydration affects the body and how forgoing water might increase our mother's pain. If we turned her now, we needed to do so with the utmost care.

"You can lessen the effects of dehydration with a gel we call 'Hospice Mix.'"

"You mean the green stuff?" we asked.

"That's another name for it," said the nurse, and we all laughed.

"It's one third mineral oil, one third KY jelly – the plain kind – and one third mouthwash, preferably without alcohol."

The nurse held up a little stick with a pink sponge on the end. "If you dip this into the green stuff and swab your mother's mouth, you'll reduce her sensation of thirst."

We thought of the dry beast in the shadows of her room, and we swallowed hard.

"Your mother's blood pressure is dropping," said the nurse. "And she appears to be anxious. She's trying to stay alert so she can talk to you."

We nodded. We so wanted to hear her words.

The nurse's voice was gentle. "You can help her move toward death by keeping the room very calm and very still."

How long, we asked. How long will she be with us?

"Three to five more days," said the nurse.

Shortly after dinner, Good Moon's nephew arrived from an ancient city in the Far East.

Good Moon looked at the man standing by her bed. "Hello," she said. "Thank you for coming."

Did she recognize the Traveller? It wasn't clear.

"I've had a glorious day," she said.

"Good Moon had a call today on her new iPhone," said the Constant One. "On Skype!"

"You must be using the iPhone 4," said the Traveller.

"No," said Good Moon, "I have an iPhone 4s. I have a nephew who works in the Far East. His company makes components for the iPhone 4s."

"Your nephew is here now," said the Constant One.

Good Moon stared at the Traveller. Her nephew? Was it possible? And then she smiled. "I can't believe you're here."

The Traveller sat down on the bed. "I've come to celebrate with you. On the plane, I read about a newly discovered planet, Kepler 22B." His voice ignited, energised. "It's 600 million light years away, so it will take an unfathomable amount of time to get there."

Good Moon's eyes were bright. She loved outer space.

"The scientists who discovered the planet found two black holes at the same time," said the Traveller. "They are hundreds of times larger than anything we've ever imagined."

"I recently saw a program on string theory," said Good Moon.

At these words, the Traveller wept. Good Moon shared his love of all that was unknown. How could he bear this loss?

"Your life has been full of adventures," said the Traveller. "This will be your next destination. When you get there, please let me know where you are."

"I will," said Good Moon. "I will ring a bell."

That evening, the Artisan leaned over her mother to say good night.

"We'll read stories tomorrow," said Good Moon.

The Artisan went to the living room and sat on the rug with her back against the sofa. She needed something strong to hold herself in place.

And then – at the core of her skull – explosive pain. An eruption of wings. Sharp, blinding, bone-white pain.

The owl, thought the Artisan. Death's voyageur. Good Moon was on her way.

2014 ©Two Ravens Pty Limited.

After a time, the Artisan dried her eyes. She looked beyond, went searching for the owl. When she found it, the owl was faring well. It knew the way. Its wings moved silently across the dark of the universe, like the breath of a sleeping child.

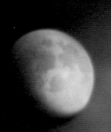

DAY FIVE, THURSDAY

GREY LAND

GOOD MOON WOKE at sunrise and turned toward the Constant One. "I've been thinking," she said.

"What have you been thinking?" asked the Constant One.

"I've been thinking about learning to Skype on my mobile."

Later that morning, Good Moon's children and grandchildren sat in the dining room.

The nurse from Hospice explained that the odour in the sun room – a slightly bitter, acidic smell – was the scent of a body moving toward death.

"Your mother's level of oxygen is dropping," said the nurse. "She's undergoing a dramatic change in her level of consciousness. Your mother's interaction with you is waning. She will spend more and more time sleeping."

We nodded. We understood.

"Even if your mother appears to be comatose," the nurse continued, "she'll be able to hear you. When you're with her, what you say to her – and about her – will matter. She'll be able to hear you, even if she can't speak to you or signal that she's here with us.

"As your mother approaches her death, your role is to keep the room as quiet as possible. Try not to pull her back. Your mother is exactly where she needs to be."

The nurse looked at each of us. She appeared to be counting heads, making sure that none of us was lost along the way.

As she left, she said, "I live so far in the grey land."

And then it was afternoon.

Good Moon's children and grandchildren sat around the dining room table, addressing Good Moon's Christmas cards. When the Artisan came in with her cello, everyone groaned.

"We don't want to be hard on you," said the Laughing One, "but you haven't been playing that long. We don't want the noise to kill Good Moon." Everyone laughed. "If the sound is too awful, we'll have to ask you to stop."

The Artisan went into the sun room and leaned over Good Moon's bed. "I'm going to play for you on my cello. My siblings have said that, if it's too bad, they're going to intervene. They don't want me to kill you."

Good Moon smiled.

In the glow of the December sun, the Artisan played for her mother, ending with "As the deer longs after the water brook, so longeth my soul for thee, O Lord."

It had been well over twenty four hours since Good Moon had taken her last ice chip. Although we had been swabbing her mouth with the green stuff, she was very, very thirsty.

The Artisan played and thought about the ancestors. There they were, at the edge of the universe, standing around a cistern of cool water. An ancient elder was looking across the darkness toward a fragment of light, the tip of a snow-white wing, just visible. In his hand was a ladle so full of liquid that it spilled over the edge in a waterfall.

"It was beautiful," said Good Moon. "Play it again."

The Artisan began to play. This time, Good Moon raised her arms and conducted.

As the sun began to set, Good Moon said, "I want to see my sons."

The Penitent leaned over the bed. "I'm here now."

Good Moon looked up at him. "I didn't want it to be like this."

"It's okay," said the Penitent. "God has called you."

"I never thought it would be this sad and this poignant."

"It is incredibly sad," said the Penitent, "but it's also incredibly joyful."

The Penitent thought of a haiku he had written. He spoke quietly, next to his mother's ear:

> Silent winter's night
> Wolves side by side through the trees
> Blue-lit braided lake

"The haiku describes a moonlit night in winter," he said. "The wolves are your family. We are walking with you through the forest until we emerge at the edge of a frozen lake. We step onto the lake and leave behind us braided trails. We are by your side as you make the crossing."

A winter landscape opened before the Penitent's eyes. "When we reach the far shore, the dark trees rise to meet us, but beyond them, there is light."

The Penitent looked further still. "And then you leave us. There is a narrow trail into the pines, and you walk on, alone. The trail widens, and the trees and the land, the sun and the moon and the stars – they all open up."

There were tears in Good Moon's eyes. "It's so peaceful," she said. "I don't know why I'm crying."

39

Later that evening, the Witness and the Fledgling came to sit with Good Moon. She lifted her hands and rubbed them against the whiskers of her son and grandson.

"We will tell this story to our children, and they will tell it to their children," said the Fledgling. "How Good Moon proceeded on her journey."

Good Moon turned toward the Fledgling. "It's so peaceful," she said. "There should be more written about this."

"Written about what?" asked the Fledgling

"About dying like this, at home."

The Fledgling nodded. "Is it good?"

"It's wonderful," said Good Moon.

The Fledgling thought about his grandmother's words. "You've inspired an idea – a biography of a woman who is dying. As she approaches her death, she uses fewer and fewer words."

And the woman's last words? What would they be?

"The last words," said the Fledgling. "They are – the most interesting – and complex."

Good Moon looked up at her grandson. "The fewer the words said, the fewer the words that need to be said."

More children and grandchildren came into the sun room. They held a star over Good Moon's bed and sang:

> Twinkle, twinkle little star
> How I wonder what you are
> Up above the world so high
> Like a diamond in the sky.
> Twinkle, twinkle little star
> How I wonder what you are.

And then, together, "We love you." And then, one after the other, "Good night, Good Moon."

An hour later, Good Moon slipped into wakefulness. With the Penitent holding the flashlight, the Artisan read *Goodnight Moon.*

When the Artisan came to the scene with the grandmother sitting in the rocker, she read:

> And a quiet old lady who was whispering "hush"
> Goodnight room
> Goodnight moon
> Goodnight cow jumping over the moon

Good Moon smiled.

Shortly thereafter, the Driver arrived from the far north.

When Good Moon heard the voice of her youngest child, she called to him and reached out to touch him.

She asked for the doors of the sun room to be opened wide. The Driver was here, and she wanted to hear the laughter of her children.

Yes, laughter.

At first, we weren't so sure. We knew that we could cry, crack in half from grief. We expected these emotions. Anger, too. We wanted her to live.

But the rest of it? Could we still tease each other? Continue telling jokes? Poke each other in the ribs? Carry on as we always had? Enjoy ourselves with dying just a room away?

We did it – all of it. We needed to, and, somehow, it was right. We were the living, and we lived.

We gathered in the living room and listened to the Driver's stories. Some were new, but most were old, and we knew the old ones by heart. We listened and laughed until we wept. Our souls were dry, and they began to fill.

The Driver told us the one about Good Moon's carrot soup, a watery sludge that was filled with slimy, floating things.

“What to do?” said the Driver. “So I took the soup out to the laundry room. You know, I felt bad about that –”

“Sure you did,” we laughed.

“All right,” said the Driver. “Not that bad. I looked around. I didn’t want her to see me. Then I poured the soup down the drain, and I told her it was great.”

Years later, we could hear the soup splashing in the sink, struggling with the drain.

We didn’t want the story to end. We were still so dry.

“Was it a cold soup?” we wanted to know.

“No,” said the Driver. “It was orange.”

♦♦

The Artisan listened to the laughter and thought about the One from Far Away. He was one of Good Moon’s sons, the brother who could not be there. He had sent a note.

The Artisan thought about her brother’s words, his own encounter with cancer some twenty years before:

> I am not able to be with you in your time of need, but this is my wish for you. I was scared and all alone. They wheeled me down the long corridor before my surgery. It was dark, quiet. It was the end. Then I remembered a portion of the Psalm of David: “Even though I walk through the valley of the shadow of death, I shall fear no evil, for Thou art with me.”

2014 ©Two Ravens Pty Limited.

The Artisan recalled that day, remembered her fear for her brother's life. But he had survived. He was with them still, though far away.

Her brother's note had ended with a prayer:

> It is when you reach this point that I pray for a miracle for you – anything, anything at all in which you feel the power of your God. Put out your hand to Him. It will be okay.

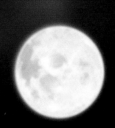

DAY SIX, FRIDAY

EXPERIMENT

FREE Gift ~ Your Choice:

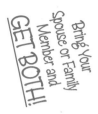

Bring Your
Spouse or Family
Member and
GET BOTH!

FREE Turkey Certificate*

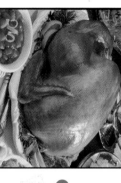

or

**FREE Honey Glazed
Ham Certificate***

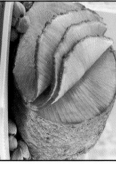

Present This Insert During Your FREE, NO OBLIGATION Hearing Exam *

*Limit one certificate per family except for accompanying family member. Hearing evaluation must be completed and must show 40db loss to receive free certificate. New customers only. Does not apply to prior purchases. Gift certificates are good toward the purchase of Butterball turkeys or many other brands of your choice. Offer valid during open house dates only.

If You Already Own Hearing Aids Receive...

Lifetime Service Guarantee & FREE unlimited Office Visits Forever

A FREE Gift From Miracle-Ear

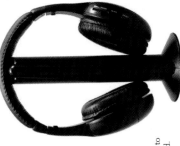

As our way of saying thanks for stopping by and allowing us to test your hearing, you will receive a **FREE** set of TV ListenEars.*

Call today, quantities are limited to stock in the office!

Please bring a spouse, family member, or a friend with you for the familiar voice portion of the evaluation. FREE offer available to new candidates who complete a hearing test.* Limit one per household.

Offer valid during open house dates only.
*Must complete hearing test & show 40db loss in order to receive FREE TV ListenEars. Limit one per household. See office for details.

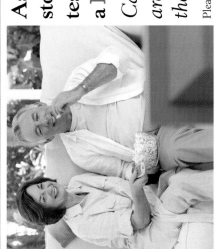

ℳ Miracle-Ear®

70147

IN THE EARLY HOURS of the morning, the Laughing One went to check on her mother. She sat on the bed and held Good Moon's hand in her own.

Good Moon reached for her daughter, and the Laughing One laid her head on her mother's breast. She felt the beating of Good Moon's heart, and in the depth of her grief she wept in her mother's arms.

"I wish I could go with you," said the Laughing One.

"We'll have to work on that," said Good Moon.

The Laughing One was asleep on the floor of the sun room when she woke to the sound of her mother's voice. It was 3 am, and the room was bathed in moonlight.

The Laughing One looked out the window. "Can you see the moon?"

"No," said Good Moon. "Please move my bed."

The Laughing One eyed the brakes on the bed and tried to release the one closest to her. She pulled and she pushed, and she pushed and she pulled, but nothing happened.

The Constant One came in and tried the brake. "Student nurses," she sighed. "They always jam the brakes."

As tired as she was, the Laughing One began to laugh.

"There she goes again," said the Constant One, and Good Moon smiled.

With one swift movement, the Constant One released the brake and steered the bed toward the window. The Laughing One lifted Good Moon's head toward the sky.

A cool blue light drifted onto the bed, and Good Moon's hair turned a translucent white. The Cold Moon – December's moon – was nearly full.

"Is the moon calming you?" asked the Laughing One.

"No," said Good Moon.

Good Moon slept until sunrise.

When the Laughing One looked in on her, Good Moon's eyes were open. She spoke slowly, but her mind was clear. "The reason and purpose for my dying," she said, "are to understand the importance of water." She went on to describe the depth of her thirst.

The Constant One came in to moisten her mother's mouth. She rubbed the swab across Good Moon's lips and up, over and under her tongue.

Good Moon smiled. "It's so good."

"Do you want something to return you to a dreamy state?" asked the Constant One.

"But what about my experiment?"

Experiment? What experiment? But there was no time to ask. Good Moon was racing on.

"I am basically happy," she said. "My purpose in life was to be a problem solver."

"Speaking of problems," said the Constant One, "the Witness is here. He was in the newspaper yesterday."

Good Moon wanted to hear the story. The Witness told of entrepreneurs with big plans. Environmentalists in opposition. The government in the middle. Too much data, too many assumptions, and far too many agendas.

Good Moon listened to her son. From time to time she asked a question. She still had one foot in this world.

"At the end of the day," said the Witness, "we ran their assumptions through the models, and we have confidence in our assumptions. "

Good Moon smiled. "I'll bet it's hard not to tell them, 'I told you so.'"

Later that day, the nurse from Hospice explained that the dying often experience a surge, one last burst of energy, before they drift into a final coma.

That rich, thoughtful discussion with Good Moon was, we believe, her last great effort. After that, her words came to us in fragments, a mosaic almost complete.

Good Moon's daughters gathered in the living room.

"What I can't get my head around is the speed," said the Artisan. "How it happened so fast."

"When Good Moon received the final diagnosis," said the Constant One, "we think she made a decision to stop eating."

The Artisan tried to absorb this thought. "What has she eaten?"

"Half a cracker and a couple of bites of egg – a week ago Wednesday," said the Constant One. "As you know, Good Moon underwent a huge surgery. She came through it beautifully, but afterward she was in a weakened state. In these circumstances, if you choose not to eat, you can hasten your death."

"I see," said the Artisan.

No food for nearly a week and a half. No water for the past two days. Good Moon didn't want to die from cancer. She wanted to die from Death. That was the experiment.

The Laughing One went into the sun room. Good Moon's arm was reaching toward the sky. She appeared to be waving at someone.

Gently, ever so gently, the Laughing One returned her mother's arm to earth.

Good Moon woke an hour later. "May I please have a glass of water?"

The Constant One ran the swab around Good Moon's mouth, across her lips, and up, over and under her tongue. Once. Twice. Three times.

Good Moon waved her arm, and the Laughing One asked, "What do you need?"

"I'm giving you the keys," said Good Moon.

"What are they for?"

"I don't know."

The Laughing One raised her hand and plucked Good Moon's keys from the air. "I have your keys. Thank you."

Just before noon, Good Moon's sons came to sit with her.

"We're going to teach your youngest – the Driver – how to swab your mouth," said the Penitent.

"That will be a pretty difficult project," said the Witness, "but we'll give it a shot."

The brothers laughed, and Good Moon smiled. "You guys are so cute."

In the early afternoon, the Witness sat with Good Moon. Saying little, seeing much, he held Good Moon deep in his heart.

He thought back to his last journey with Good Moon, a canoe trip in the land of the voyageurs. Good Moon and the Witness had driven north along the shores of the great lake. At one point, a grey shadow had crossed in front of the car. A wolf, vanishing into the trees like a mist.

Mother and son had traversed the far north and had talked for hours and hours. At the end of the trip, Good Moon had said, "I will not be coming here again."

Midway through the afternoon, we sat with the nurse from Hospice.

"Your mother has a far away, glazed look," said the nurse. "It's as if she's looking through us rather than at us. We call this 'the time of transitioning.'

"To pull her back would create a lot of stress. We encourage you to talk but not to ask questions. If you need to care for her, tell her in advance what you plan to do."

The nurse looked at us and saw the question in our eyes. How long now?

"An educated guess would be 24 to 48 hours," said the nurse. "She's not fully here, and she's not fully there. Most of the time, she will not be lucid. She'll be sleeping."

We nodded. We had seen the change.

"Her levels of oxygen and responsiveness and her vital signs have all declined," said the nurse. "But right now she is very comfortable. She has a beautiful, glowing smile. She's on the right level of medication, and that will keep the pain from coming back."

The nurse explained how the dying breathe. "If your mother makes a gurgling sound, please don't worry. We call it 'fish out of water breathing.' She's not in distress. It's simply a bodily function – the diaphragm is spasming. It's completely normal, and she will not be in pain.

"There may be times when she won't breathe at all. Try not to breathe with her."

The nurse held her breath, and when at last she gasped for air, we burst out laughing. Without knowing it, we had held our breath as well.

"You need to put drops of saline in her eyes to keep them moist," said the nurse. "During this time, her eyes may open, and they may stay open. The same with her mouth. Your mother may die that way – with her mouth and her eyes open.

"That peaceful look in the movies? It's often not there." And then, gently. "The body will try much harder than the soul to stay."

Later that afternoon, Sapphire sat in the sun room with her grandmother. "You're surrounded by purple," said Sapphire. "Such good energy." "I prefer blue," said Good Moon.

As the sun began to set, the doctor came by the house.
Good Moon said, "You would be an angel to get me a glass of water."

At twilight, the Constant One spoke to her mother. "Good Moon, you can go. You can leave me. I have my daughter, my friends and the Laughing One. They will take care of me."

Good Moon raised her hand and held up three fingers. "Scout's honour?"

"Scout's honour," said the Constant One.

After dinner, we changed Good Moon's bedding, and we gave her a bath. All of us were there. Together, we lifted our mother as if to place her on a magic carpet.

Good Moon said, "It feels really good."

Although we didn't know it at the time, these were her last words.

DAY SEVEN, SATURDAY

TOTAL ECLIPSE

WE WOKE ON SATURDAY to a total eclipse of the moon.

As we were in the heartland, far from the ocean, the eclipse would be nearly invisible. If we were lucky, the moon would just skirt the edge of the horizon.

The Artisan went outside to look for the moon. The sky was empty. It was grey and clear, and there was nothing there.

The Artisan looked again, this time beyond, and then she saw it. A broken arc of cool blue light.

As the eclipse approached totality, the Laughing One said to her mother, "I'm behind you on this journey."

Good Moon's eyes opened and closed.

"I'm so proud of you," said the Laughing One. "Go be with the angels."

At midmorning, we met in the sun room.

"Good Moon," said the Witness. "We're going to do your morning care."

Good Moon's eyes opened. A moment later, they closed.

"We're going to lift you," said the Witness, "and we're going to change you. All of us are here."

We gathered around the bed, and each of us slid our hands under Good

Moon's body – her head, her upper back, her arms, her legs. And then we flinched. Good Moon's face had filled with pain.

As soon as she was airborne, the pain vanished as quickly as it had come. Good Moon's face returned to calm.

That was hard for us – cleansing the nest and disturbing the rest of our elder.

We checked on Good Moon throughout the day, but she did not wake up.

In the afternoon, the Constant One spoke to Good Moon and gave her medication. Good Moon's eyes flickered.

After that Good Moon's eyes were closed, and they did not open again.

Of all eight days, Saturday was the hardest. We wanted Good Moon to stay with us forever. And we needed her to die.

We were, like her, in the grey land, deep in the shadows of a world that wasn't ours. When we spoke, we had no breath. When we walked, the earth disappeared beneath our feet. We could not laugh, and we could not dream. We wandered through the house, aimless and out of life. Our souls were tired from the strain of death.

We had gone with her as far as we could go, and we needed to move on. We needed her to leave.

When we realised that we had changed, that we were letting go, we cringed. We wished that we were different, that dying were different.

We wanted Good Moon to speak to us with her final breath, to live, as we were living, up to the very end. Instead, we were met with silence, a body flat on the bed, eyes closed, mouth open, breathing.

Late in the day, the nurse from Hospice sat with us one last time.

"Your mother's level of oxygen is very low," said the nurse. "She could die at any time."

The nurse looked at the Constant One. "Your sister, with your support, is doing a great job of keeping her comfortable. Your mother's blood pressure and pulse rate are higher than I would have expected, so she may be experiencing discomfort. We may need to increase her medication."

We tried to absorb these words.

"Your mother is in tune with the moon," said the nurse. "It creates a different atmospheric pressure right before dawn." She spoke to us as gently as she could. "The dying tend to leave us in the middle of the night. On their own time."

DAY EIGHT, SUNDAY

SKY BURIAL

SUNDAY BEGAN AT MIDNIGHT for Good Moon's daughters. We made beds for ourselves on the floor of the sun room. We did not want our mother to die alone.

The Constant One had seen many births and many deaths, and we asked her to help us understand.

"I think what we have now is a shell – that Good Moon's spirit left us earlier today." The Constant One looked at us thoughtfully. "That's just my opinion. No one knows, of course."

"Why do you think that?" asked the Artisan.

"It has to do with the waxiness of her skin. And her breathing. Earlier in the day, Good Moon breathed as if she were asleep. Now she sounds like a machine."

We listened to our mother breathe. What we heard was her diaphragm, the machine beneath, pumping air into her body. The sound was mechanical, even, hollow, and there was a rasp to it, as if she needed oil.

The Artisan offered to keep the first watch. She lay on the floor between her sisters and listened to a body trying to hold onto life.

Deep in the night, Sleep tiptoed into the room. The Artisan checked her watch. It was 4 am.

Ah, Good Moon, she thought. You're watching over your daughters. You want us to fall asleep so that you can slip away.

Isn't that what the nurse from Hospice had said – that mothers die alone so they don't bring pain to their children?

59

The Constant One took the next watch. At the first promise of dawn, she woke her sisters. "Good Moon is breathing more slowly."

"We need to get our brothers," said the Artisan.

We gathered blankets, sleeping bags and pillows, and we lay on the floor of the sun room. We left ample space around Good Moon. We did not want to crowd an elder in her nest.

That morning, we drank our coffee in the sun room.

The Constant One and the Laughing One sat on the bed. They took turns reading notes from Good Moon's many friends.

The Witness pulled up a chair and sat with a notepad on his lap. He would give the eulogy, and from time to time, he wrote down a phrase.

Everyone else sat on the floor.

"Good Moon didn't want a vigil," said the Constant One.

"Then we'll have to call this something else," said the Artisan. "How about morning coffee?"

Later, we learned that the moon had set at 8:35 am.

The Artisan looked out the window. A small songbird flitted by. Brown and non-descript, it skittered across the sky and disappeared.

Then – something.

"A big, dark bird is circling out there," said the Artisan. "Does anyone know what it is?"

"Is it really big?" asked the Witness.

"It's really big," said the Artisan.

"Then it's a raven." The Witness stood up to confirm the sighting. "There are two."

We watched them soar over the trees. They were huge. Their dark wings flashed and covered the sky with a shroud, a presence beyond the land of the living.

The first raven paused overhead, and then it flew away. The second one landed on the tree across the street. It sat on the topmost bough, facing us.

"Ravens are very, very smart," said the Witness. "They sense death."

"The Tibetans lay their dead on a rocky slope," said the Artisan. "The vultures come and pick the bones clean. Good Moon said once that the Tibetan ritual made great sense to her."

"They call it a 'sky burial,'" said the Penitent.

We sat under the watchful eye of the raven as the dark presence gathered around us.

The Constant One counted breaths as she had so many times before. "I think we're getting close."

Good Moon's children rose and circled the bed, their arms around each other.

The Artisan looked out the window. The raven unfurled its wings, took flight, and vanished.

"That was her last breath," said the Constant One.

We waited for the next breath, which did not come.

He stood where he always stood, with the ancestors at the edge of the universe, next to the cistern, ladle in hand, ready with water.

He looked toward earth. Below, a family circled an empty bed, silent in the face of death.

He turned his ancient eyes from earth and looked across the dark. The fragment of light was now an owl – large, white-winged and amber-eyed. On its back was a woman's soul.

He smiled. He knew her name.

Turn right, Good Moon, he said. Turn right.

After - Mosaic

When Good Moon said that more should be written about dying at home, and when she told us she was pleased that we were writing down our conversations with her, we believed that we had her blessing to share her last days with others.

Looking back, we believe that dying at home was what Good Moon wanted, and we were fortunate enough to be able to fulfill her wish. Nevertheless, as we learned during the final days of her life, "dying at home" was quite a complex undertaking, something that required many skilled hands – and many hands other than ours – to bring to fruition.

We are grateful to our sister, the Constant One, who brought her deep knowledge and professionalism to the nursing of our mother. During her years as a nurse, our sister had witnessed many deaths. Her familiarity and level of comfort with dying gave us solace and security. The Constant One and her husband opened their home to us, and we benefited throughout from their gracious hospitality and willingness to make their home ours.

The "nurse from Hospice" is a composite of three nurses, each of whom brought her unique wisdom to our mother's last days. We are deeply grateful to these nurses for sharing their many years of experience with us. We are also grateful to the doctor who visited our mother and worked with us to keep her level of pain as low as possible.

My mother and we were blessed with the spiritual guidance of two men of faith – the Dakotan holy man who named our mother Wasté Hanyetuwi and the Methodist pastor who prayed with us when our mother decided to forgo further liquid. Their kind words and connection to the next world filled us with joy and calm, helping to balance our sorrow.

The Constant One had many friends who shared their homes with us so that we could stay in the neighbourhood, near our mother. These friends cooked for us. They shopped and ran errands and provided care for our mother. They laughed with us. And they held us when we cried. We give thanks in particular to Dragonfly, who sensed our needs before we even knew we had them.

Good Moon had a large family. We are grateful to the many relatives who travelled great distances to be with her, and we thank all members of the family, including our father, for supporting Good Moon on her journey.

An artisan cannot create a mosaic without pieces of many different colours. I am deeply grateful to my brothers and sisters for their willingness to share their conversations with Good Moon. Because we journeyed together, each of us was less alone with our grief, and we were able to give each other comfort through the word-raft that Good Moon helped us build.

Finally, I am fortunate to have met and worked with a fine designer who was able to translate what we saw into a visual frame to hold our story. I know that Good Moon, were she to hold this small volume in her hands, would smile.